Health and Medical Trivia

Lance D. Williams

Published by Lance D. Williams, 2023.

HEALTH AND MEDICAL TRIVIA

First edition. July 22, 2023.

ISBN: 979-8223132479

Written by Lance D. Williams.

Table of Contents

(Introduction)

I wanted to do this type of trivia so people would learn more about things they may not know about. Breast cancer is talked about all the time, but there are more than 200 different types of cancer that don't get talked about. I used to be the type of person who didn't care about eating unhealthy food if it was delicious. But when I finally started paying attention to what really goes into the food, beverages, and products I bought and learning how corporations, the FDA, and other people and places in charge allow so many harmful things in our society, I took it more seriously, especially as a parent and not wanting to do more harm to my kids.

In my early years as a parent, I would buy them McDonald's or Subway, let them eat Skittles, and drink soda. Starting their day off with sugary cereal, oatmeal, and unhealthy yogurt. It can really be a wake-up call when you start to research the ingredients in products, like GMOs and Roundup Weed Killer residue in food and even the water we drink and shower with is harmful in many areas without filters.

There are different types of disorders and injuries that most people don't know about. So, like I do on a regular basis, I like to research and learn new things, then I pass it on to my kids so they can learn, and then I make it a book so other people can learn as well.

(Chapter 1)

1- Which one is a rare form of gynecologic cancer?

(A)- Metastatic Cancer

(B)- Fallopian Tube Cancer

(C)- Colorectal Cancer

(D)- Oral Cancer

2- The most common cause of dementia is ...

(A)- Huntington's Disease

(B)- Alzheimer's Disease

(C)- Brain Tumor

(D)- Chronic Traumatic Encephalopathy

3- When a bone cracks on one side only, not all the way through the bone, it is called ...

(A)- Plantar Fasciitis

(B)- Achilles Tendonitis

(C)- Sesamoiditis

(D)- Greenstick Fracture

4- Which one is a rare, progressive neurological disorder?

(A)- Spina Bifida

(B)- Intervertebral Disc Degeneration

(C)- Neurofibromatosis

(D)- Stiff-Person Syndrome

5- This contains trans-fat, which is strongly correlated with an increased risk of type 2 diabetes and heart disease.

(A)- Carrageenan

(B)- Polysorbate 80

(C)- Mono and Diglycerides

(D)- Glyphosate

6- Many people hear a pop or feel a popping sensation in the knee when this injury occurs.

(A)- Lateral Cruciate Ligament (LCL)

(B)- Posterior Cruciate Ligament (PCL)

(C)- Anterior Cruciate Ligament (ACL)

(D)- Medial Collateral Ligament (MCL)

7- This inherited condition causes hundreds, and sometimes thousands of abnormal growths throughout the body.

(A)- Appendicitis

(B)- Hyperthyroidism

(C)- Gardner's Syndrome

(D)- Inguinal Hernia

8- Which one is classified as a motor neuron disease?

(A)- Spinal Muscular Atrophy

(B)- Fetal Alcohol Syndrome

(C)- Urinary Tract Infection (UTI)

(D)- Tay-Sachs Disease

9- This is known as a swallowing disorder.

(A)- Strep throat

(B)- Acute Bronchitis

(C)- Tonsillitis

(D)- Dysphagia

10- Which one is a chemotherapy drug?

(A)- Podophyllotoxin

(B)- Mercaptopurine

(C)- Listeria Monocytogenes

(D)- Antimetabolites

11- In the 1970s, this was banned.

(A)- Potassium Bromate

(B)- Propylparaben

(C)- Red Dye #2

(D)- Red Dye #3

12- Which one is known as a sleep study?

(A)- Parasomnias

(B)- Sleep Apnea

(C)- Somnambulism

(D)- Polysomnography

13- Hypertension is also known as ...

(A)- Angina

(B)- Umbilical Hernia

(C)- Heart Valve Disease

(D)- High Blood Pressure

14- This often occurs when the stool is hardened, and people have been constipated for a long time.

(A)- Irritable Bowel Syndrome

(B)- Short Bowel Syndrome (SBS)

(C)- Fecal Impaction

(D)- Anal Fissure

15- This is known as tennis elbow.

(A)- Lateral Epicondylitis

(B)- Medial Epicondylitis

(C)- Rhuematoid Arthritis

(D)- Olecranon Bursitis

(Chapter 1) Answers

1- B

2- B

3- D

4- D

5- C

6- C

7- C

8- A

9- D

10- B

11- C

12- D

13- D

14- C

15- A

(Chapter 2)

16- This is a disease that is associated with dysfunction of the proximal tubule of the kidney.

(A)- Fanconi Syndrome

(B)- Down Syndrome

(C)- Proteus Syndrome

(D)- Tourette Syndrome

17- What is known as sugar alcohol?

(A)- Formaldehyde

(B)- Erythritol

(C)- Monsodium Glutamate (MSG)

(D)- Phthalates

18- This is the 5th most common GI cancer in the United States.

(A)- Parathyroid Cancer

(B)- Testicular Cancer

(C)- Gallbladder Cancer

(D)- Uterine Cancer

19- People with this have an irrational fear of gaining weight and put themselves on restrictive diets that can cause severe health issues.

(A)- Bulimia Nervosa

(B)- Anorexia Nervosa

(C)- Binge-Eating Disorder (BED)

(D)- Avoidant Restrictive Food Intake Disorder (ARFID)

20- This is severe scarring of the liver.

(A)- Polycystic Kidney Disease

(B)- Cirrhosis

(C)- Pancreatitis

(D)- Gastroesophageal Reflux Disease

21- Swollen, inflamed veins around the anus and lower part of the rectum is called ...

(A)- Microscopic Colitis

(B)- Crohn's Disease

(C)- Hemorrhoids

(D)- Colon Polyps

22- This is a milder form of bipolar disorder.

(A)- Chronic Fatigue Syndrome

(B)- Wernicke Aphasia

(C)- Cyclothymia

(D)- Pheochromocytoma

23- Which one is spread to people through the bite of an infected Aedes species?

(A)- Human Immunodeficiency Virus

(B)- Monkeypox Virus

(C)- Dengue Virus

(D)- Human Papillomavirus

24- This is usually triggered by a traumatic event, sudden stress, or a major life change.

(A)- Persistent Depressive Disorder

(B)- Seasonal Affective Disorder

(C)- Postpartum Depression

(D)- Situational Depression

25- This is an inflammatory process that causes a blood clot to form and block one or more veins, usually in the legs.

(A)- Femur Shaft Fractures

(B)- Posterior Tibial Tendon Dysfuction

(C)- Buerger's Disease

(D)- Thrombophlebitis

26- This is an inflammatory disease caused when the immune system attacks its own tissues.

(A)- Cannabis Intoxication

(B)- Lupus

(C)- Enuresis

(D)- Chronic Obstructive Pulmonary Disease (COPD)

27- This is an anxiety disorder that often develops after one or more panic attacks.

(A)- Hypochondriac

(B)- Agoraphobia

(C)- Schizophrenia

(D)- Kleptomania

28- Whooping cough is also called ...

(A)- Salmonella

(B)- Leptospirosis

(C)- Anthrax

(D)- Pertussis

29- This is a serious autoimmune disease that occurs in genetically predisposed people. It is estimated to affect 1 in 100 people worldwide.

(A)- Wilson's Disease

(B)- Parkinson's Disease

(C)- Lyme Disease

(D)- Celiac Disease

30- Which one affects the parotid glands, salivary glands below and in front of the ears?

(A)- Mumps

(B)- Giardiasis

(C)- Seizures

(D)- Cytomegalovirus

(Chapter 2) Answers

16- A

17- B

18- C

19- B

20- B

21- C

22- C

23- C

24- D

25- D

26- B

27- B

28- D

29- D

30- A

(Chapter 3)

31- This is a leading cause of death in the United States and is a major cause of serious disability for adults.

(A)- Stroke

(B)- Toxoplasmosis

(C)- Diabetes

(D)- Epstein-Barr Virus

32- A vaccine was approved by the U.S. FDA in December 2019 for this.

(A)- Coronavirus Disease 2019

(B)- Ebola Virus Disease

(C)- Smallpox

(D)- Zika Virus Infection

33- This is a condition that affects only females, when one of the X chromosomes (sex chromosomes) is missing or partially missing.

(A)- Haemochromatosis

(B)- Duchenne Muscular Dystrophy

(C)- Turner Syndrome

(D)- Cystic Fibrosis

34- This is an open sore or raw area in the lining of the stomach or intestine.

(A)- Iron Deficiency Anemia

(B)- Peptic Ulcers

(C)- Lactose Intolerance

(D)- Polycythemia Vera

35- This is also known as lazy eye.

(A)- Cataract

(B)- Glaucoma

(C)- Strabismus

(D)- Amblyopia

36- This is an acquired condition where scar tissue forms inside the uterus.

(A)- Sclerosing Adenosis

(B)- Asherman's Syndrome

(C)- Cervical Dysplasia

(D)- Fat Nerosis

37- A mental disorder in which you have thoughts and rituals over and over is called ...

(A)- Bipolar Affective Disorder

(B)- Reactive Attachment Disorder

(C)- Obsessive Compulsive Disorder

(D)- Attention Deficit Hyperactivity Disorder

38- The main symptom for bad smelling breath is ...

(A)- Receding Gums

(B)- Halitosis

(C)- Gingivitis

(D)- Root Infection

39- This occurs when the PSMB8 gene is not working correctly.

(A)- ANOTHER Syndrome

(B)- CANDLE Syndrome

(C)- DOOR Syndrome

(D)- FACES Syndrome

40- This is a fat preservative, used in foods to extend shelf life. It is linked to cancerous tumor growth.

(A)- Artificial Sweeteners

(B)- Enriched Flour

(C)- Sodium Nitrite

(D)- Butylated Hydroxyanisole

41- Which one was founded in 1947?

(A)- American Medical Women's Association

(B)- Irish College of Ophthalmologists

(C)- College of Family Physicians of Canada

(D)- British Geriatrics Society

42- This can be treated with bright light therapy or behaviorally with chronotherapy.

(A)- Colic

(B)- Liver Angiosarcoma

(C)- Advanced Sleep Phase Disorder

(D)- Cold Agglutinin Disease

43- This is also known as rabbit fever.

(A)- Clostridioides Difficile

(B)- Relapsing Fever

(C)- Tularemia

(D)- Colorado Tick Fever

44- A false pregnancy is ...

(A)- Postpartum Psychosis

(B)- Hallucinogen Persisting Perception Disorder

(C)- Munchausen Syndrome

(D)- Pseudocyesis

45- This is known as growth hormone insensitivity or growth hormone receptor deficiency.

(A)- Laron Syndrome

(B)- Weissenbacher-Zweymüller Syndrome

(C)- Knobloch Syndrome

(D)- McGillivray Syndrome

(Chapter 3) Answers

31- A

32- B

33- C

34- B

35- D

36- B

37- C

38- B

39- B

40- D

41- D

42- C

43- C

44- D

45- A

(Chapter 4)

46- Excessive uncontrollable daytime sleepiness is ...

(A)- Charcot-Marie-Tooth Disease

(B)- Trichomoniasis

(C)- Androgen Insensitivity Syndrome

(D)- Narcolepsy

47- A rare condition in which the body stops producing enough new blood cells.

(A)- Immune Thrombocytopenic Purpura

(B)- Aplastic Anemia

(C)- Sickle Cell Anemia

(D)- Acute Lymphoblastic Leukemia

48- In January 1996, the FDA approved this as a food additive.

(A)- Olestra

(B)- Yeast Extract

(C)- Guar Gum

(D)- Artificial Flavoring

49- This is a condition that occurs when small pouches, or sacs, form and push outward through weak spots in the wall of the colon.

(A)- Hirschsprung's Disease

(B)- Diverticular Disease

(C)- Barrett's Esophagus

(D)- Exocrine Pancreatic Insufficiency

50- Which one was founded in 1951?

(A)- Nigerian Medical Association

(B)- American Academy of Pediatrics

(C)- German Medical Association

(D)- European Academy of Allergy and Clinical Immunology

51- This is a condition in which a person's airways become inflamed, narrow, and swollen, and produce extra mucus making it difficult to breathe.

(A)- Emphysema

(B)- Carbon Monoxide Poisoning

(C)- Pleurisy

(D)- Asthma

52- Highly aggressive and difficult-to-treat brain tumors found at the base of the brain is ...

(A)- Scheuermann's Disease

(B)- Diffuse Intrinsic Pontine Glioma

(C)- Scoliosis

(D)- Delayed Sleep Phase Syndrome

53- A painful collection of pus is usually caused by a bacterial infection.

(A)- Abrasion

(B)- Abscess

(C)- Atrial Fibrillation

(D)- Aneurysm

54- Exomphalos is also known as ...

(A)- Polydactyly

(B)- Omphalocele

(C)- Monosomy

(D)- Abortive Polio

55- A deadly virus that spreads to people from the saliva of infected animals is ....

(A)- Color Blindness

(B)- Usher Syndrome

(C)- Rabies

(D)- Persistent Vegetative State

56- A sudden weakness in the muscles on one half of the face is ....

(A)- Progressive Supranuclear Palsy

(B)- Creutzfeldt-Jakob Disease

(C)- Bell's Palsy

(D)- Sydenham's Chorea

57- This is a substance found in all tobacco products and some e-cigarette liquids.

(A)- Methadone

(B)- Preservatives

(C)- Nicotine

(D)- Zinc Sulfate

58- A baby born with an underdeveloped brain and an incomplete skull.

(A)- Cleft Lip

(B)- Anencephaly

(C)- Fragile X Syndrome

(D)- Cerebral Palsy

59- This can happen suddenly and last for a short time, it usually happens after trauma or major stress.

(A)- Brief Psychotic Disorder

(B)- Male Menopause

(C)- Depression

(D)- Alcohol Use Disorder

60- This is traditionally used to color dairy products like natural cheddar cheese, yogurt, dairy drinks, and ice cream.

(A)- Sucralose

(B)- Camauba Wax

(C)- Propyl Gallate

(D)- Norbixin

(Chapter 4) Answers

46- D

47- B

48- A

49- A

50- A

51- D

52- B

53- B

54- B

55- C

56- C

57- C

58- B

59- A

60- D

(Chapter 5)

61- When one or more tumors grow in the pancreas or in the upper part of the small intestine it is ...

(A)- Zollinger-Ellison Syndrome

(B)- Cyclic Vomiting Syndrome

(C)- Viral Gastroenteritis

(D)- Gastrointestinal (GI) Bleeding

62- This condition that causes inflammation in the walls of some blood vessels in the body is ....

(A)- Cauda Equina Syndrome

(B)- Oat Cell Cancer

(C)- Kawasaki Disease

(D)- Tachycardia

63- Trimethylaminnuria is known as ...

(A)- Fish Odor Syndrome

(B)- Nail-patella Syndrome

(C)- Jadassohn-Lewandowski Syndrome

(D)- Achoo Syndrome

64- This is a partial or complete break in the bone.

(A)- Erectile Dysfunction

(B)- Fracture

(C)- Contusion

(D)- Biopsy

65- Which is the congenital condition that affects the formation of connective tissue called collagen?

(A)- Macroglossia

(B)- Jugular Foramen

(C)- Pituitary Gland

(D)- Stickler Syndrome

66- In March 2018, the European food safety authorities re-reviewed ____ and determined the research weighed in favor of no concern for causing cancer, DNA harming, or prenatal development.

(A)- Sodium Benzoate

(B)- Xanthan Gum

(C)- Carrageenan

(D)- High-Fructose Corn Syrup

67- Which is thicker than normal and often oval shaped?

(A)- Discoid Meniscus

(B)- Rotator Cuff Tear

(C)- Deep Gluteal Pain Syndrome

(D)- Bankart Lesion

68- This is a form of male birth control that cuts the supply of sperm to semen.

(A)- Chlamydia

(B)- Hip Labral Tear

(C)- Vasectomy

(D)- Ostetis Pubis

69- When there is earwax blockage it is ...

(A)- Follicular Lymphoma

(B)- Phenylketonuria

(C)- Red Ear Syndrome

(D)- Cerumen Impaction

70- This is caused by damage to the memory-storage areas of the brain.

(A)- Williams Syndrome

(B)- Dissociative Identity Disorder

(C)- Parasomnia

(D)- Retrograde Amnesia

71- A gradual thickening and tightening of tissue under the skin in the hand is ...

(A)- Aggressive Periodontitis

(B)- Paronychia

(C)- Dupuytren's Contracture

(D)- Psoriatic Arthritis

72- This is referred to as a full-thickness burn and it destroys the epidermis and dermis.

(A)- First-degree burns

(B)- Second-degree burns

(C)- Third-degree burns

(D)- Fourth-degree burns

73- This occurs mainly in Southeast Asia and spreads through eating infected raw fish.

(A)- Rickettsialpox

(B)- Bacterial Meningitis

(C)- Macrovascular Disease

(D)- Opisthorchiasis

74- This has been approved by the U.S. FDA since 1988.

(A)- Magnesium Sulphate

(B)- Agave Nectar

(C)- Acesulfame Potassium

(D)- Recombinant Bovine Growth Hormone

75- Which one has to do with the foot?

(A)- Lacrimal Bone

(B)- Tarsal Bones

(C)- Occipital Bone

(D)- Cortical Bone

(Chapter 5) Answers

61- A

62- C

63- A

64- B

65- D

66- C

67- A

68- C

69- D

70- D

71- C

72- C

73- D

74- C

75- B

(Chapter 6)

76- Which one was established in 1924?

(A)- The New England Journal of Medicine

(B)- British Journal of Hospital Medicine

(C)- Journal of Infection in Developing Countries

(D)- Journal of Clinical Investigation

77- An inflammation of the eyelid that affects the eyelashes and tear production is ...

(A)- Diplopia

(B)- Histoplasmosis

(C)- Vitreous Detachment

(D)- Blepharitis

78- A prolonged erection of the penis, usually without sexual arousal is ...

(A)- Priapism

(B)- Boutonnière Deformity

(C)- Lichen Planus

(D)- Tracheoesophageal Fistula

79- This is excessive hair growth anywhere on the body in males or females.

(A)- Hyperhidrosis

(B)- Trichotillomania

(C)- Dermatophagia

(D)- Plagiocephaly

80- This is also called oculosympathetic palsy.

(A)- Photophobia

(B)- Argyll Robertson Pupils

(C)- Physiological Anisocoria

(D)- Horner's Syndrome

81- A common condition which results in enlarged male breast tissue is ...

(A)- Lambdoid Suture

(B)- Gynecomastia

(C)- Tuberous Breasts

(D)- Carpal Tunnel Syndrome

82- When someone becomes disoriented and has a change in mental abilities, it's called ...

(A)- Delirium

(B)- Fatal Familial Insomnia

(C)- Lymphatic Filariasis

(D)- Vasospasm

83- The first recorded description of the ___ was by Herophilos (335-280 BC).

(A)- Cricoid Cartilage

(B)- Hypoglossal Nerve

(C)- Submandibular Gland

(D)- Platysma Muscle

84- On August 15, 2011, this place was formed.

(A)- Brain Function Laboratory

(B)- Wisconsin National Primate Research Center

(C)- Hormel Institute

(D)- Center for Neurotechnology

85- Lip dryness, redness, cracking, and itching are common symptoms of this.

(A)- Epistaxis

(B)- Andersen Disease

(C)- Molar pregnancy

(D)- Cheilitis

86- This is a type of headache disorder. It causes constant pain in only one side of the face and head.

(A)- Frontotemporal Dementia

(B)- Hemicrania Continua

(C)- Sick Sinus Syndrome

(D)- Left Ventricular Outflow Tract Obstruction

87- This is a genetic disease that affects the skull, face, hands, and feet.

(A)- Osteosarcoma

(B)- Heliotrope Rash

(C)- Hepatocellular Carcinoma

(D)- Apert Syndrome

88- This is commonly called hot flashes and night sweats.

(A)- Vasomotor Symptoms

(B)- Kaposi's Sarcoma

(C)- Insulinoma

(D)- Mitral Valve Regurgitation

89- This is a rare disorder in which blood vessels become inflamed.

(A)- Urolagnia

(B)- Resignation Syndrome

(C)- Granulomatosis with Polyangiitis

(D)- Toxoplasmosis

90- Which one is ringing in the ears?

(A)- Vitiligo

(B)- Flaccid

(C)- Tinnitus

(D)- Amyloidsis

(Chapter 6) Answers

76- D

77- D

78- A

79- A

80- D

81- B

82- A

83- B

84- D

85- D

86- B

87- D

88- A

89- C

90- C

(Chapter 7)

91- This is a bacterial infection usually spread by sexual contact that starts as a painless sore.

(A)- Measles

(B)- Syphilis

(C)- Tuberculosis

(D)- Influenza

92- Atypical moles are also known as ...

(A)- Nodular Melanoma

(B)- Keloids

(C)- Psoriasis

(D)- Dysplastic Nevi

93- This is known as painful bladder syndrome.

(A)- Deep Vein Thrombosis

(B)- Cavernous Malformation

(C)- Interstitial Cystitis

(D)- Vesicles

94- This is a blood disorder with decreased blood platelets.

(A)- Idiopathic Thrombocytopen Purpura

(B)- Meningoencephalitis

(C)- Estrogen Insensitivity Syndrome

(D)- Vaginal Discharge

95- This occurs when the body cannot break down certain parts of the proteins found in food.

(A)- Rubinstein-Taybi Syndrome

(B)- Isovaleric Acidemia

(C)- Generalized Arterial Calcification of Infancy

(D)- Emery-Dreifuss Muscular Dystrophy

96- This is a rare skin condition that causes painful ulcers.

(A)- Lennox-Gastaut Syndrome

(B)- Mesothelioma

(C)- Pyoderma Gangrenosum

(D)- Azodicarbonamide

97- This was created in 1913.

(A)- Society of Hospital Medicine

(B)- American College of Surgeons

(C)- Urgent Care Association of America

(D)- National Association of Emergency Medical Technicians

98- When you have low amniotic fluid during pregnancy it's called ...

(A)- HELLP Syndrome

(B)- Chorioamnionitis

(C)- Oligohydraminos

(D)- Intrauterine Fetal Demise

99- This is a rare, life-shortening, neurodegenerative genetic disorder with onset occurring most in childhood.

(A)- Prolonged Grief Disorder

(B)- Cytochrome C Oxidase Deficiency

(C)- Night Eating Syndrome

(D)- Riboflavin Transporter Deficiency

100- This is a chronic disease in which the small bile ducts in the liver become injured, inflamed, and destroyed.

(A)- Primary Biliary Cholangitis

(B)- Wiskott-Aldrich Syndrome

(C)- Sacrococcygeal Teratoma

(D)- Mucosal Melanoma

101- This was established in 1982.

(A)- Primary Dental Journal

(B)- Rejuvenation Research

(C)- Statistics in Medicine

(D)- Journal of Pain Research

102- This is a condition caused by the body's inability to absorb certain protein building blocks (amino acids) from the diet.

(A)- Q fever

(B)- Vernal Keratoconjunctivitis

(C)- Hartnup Disease

(D)- Wiedemann-Rautenstrauch Syndrome

103- Bone cracking and joint popping is ...

(A)- Sequela

(B)- Crepitus

(C)- Atherosclerosis

(D)- Cushing Syndrome

104- This is a type of cancer that starts in mucus-producing (glandular) cells.

(A)- Pilocytic astrocytoma

(B)- Dermatillomania

(C)- Adenocarcinoma

(D)- Root Canal

105- What is it called when there's an irregularly fast or erratic heartbeat?

(A)- Fibrolamellar hepatocellular carcinoma

(B)- Gelineau Syndrome

(C)- Scabies

(D)- Supraventricular Tachycard

(Chapter 7) Answers

91- B

92- D

93- C

94- A

95- B

96- C

97- B

98- C

99- D

100- A

101- C

102- C

103- B

104- C

105- D

(Chapter 8)

106- In 1966, this was listed as an approved food dye by the U.S. FDA.

(A)- Red #40

(B)- Orange B

(C)- Titanium Dioxide

(D)- Blue #1

107- This is known as werewolf syndrome?

(A)- Tinea Corporis

(B)- Fascioliasis

(C)- Hypotrichosis

(D)- Duchenne Muscular Dystrophy

108- One case of this disease is found in every 250,000 to 600,000 babies.

(A)- Leydig Cell Tumor

(B)- Schimke Immuno-Osseous Dysplasia

(C)- Maroteaux-Lamy Syndrome

(D)- Respiratory Syncytial Virus

109- According to the National Library of Medicine, studies found this to cause liver enlargement, neurotoxic effects, convulsions, and paralysis in laboratory animals.

(A)- Disodium Inosinate

(B)- tert-Butylhydroquinone

(C)- Aluminum

(D)- Propylene Glycol

110- This is a rare complex birth defect involving the urinary, reproductive, and intestinal tracts.

(A)- Bladder Exstrophy

(B)- Sudden Infant Death Syndrome

(C)- Nephrogenic Diabetes Insipidus

(D)- Smith-McCort Dysplasia

111- Firm lumps under the skin, that tend to form close to joints is called ...

(A)- Groin Pull

(B)- Ischial Bursitis

(C)- Hip Flexor Strain

(D)- Rheumatoid Nodules

112- This is also known as Silk Road disease.

(A)- Spondyloepiphyseal Dysplasia Tarda

(B)- Behçet's Syndrome

(C)- Scalp Ringworm

(D)- Paget's Disease of the Breast

113- This rare disorder involves an overgrowth of cells in your body's lymph nodes.

(A)- Reaven Syndrome

(B)- Castleman Disease

(C)- Krukenberg Tumor

(D)- Atopic Dermatitis

114- Which one is a genetic condition that results when a boy is born with an extra copy of the X chromosome?

(A)- Trisomy 13 Syndrome

(B)- Cytomegalovirus

(C)- Danon Disease

(D)- Klinefelter Syndrome

115- This bimonthly peer-reviewed medical journal was established in 1991.

(A)- Breast Cancer Research and Treatment

(B)- American Journal of Medical Genetics

(C)- Melanoma Research

(D)- Chinese Medical Journal

116- This is a skin condition that causes small blisters on the palms of hands, soles of the feet and edges of the fingers and toes.

(A)- Multiple Sclerosis

(B)- Dyshidrotic Eczema

(C)- Second-Impact Syndrome

(D)- Esthesioneuroblastoma

117- Which one was established in 1972?

(A)- Journal of Medical Case Reports

(B)- Current Medical Research and Opinion

(C)- Pan American Journal of Public Health

(D)- Biological Research for Nursing

118- This was banned in 1981 because of fear of possible carcinogenesis.

(A)- Saccharin

(B)- BHA/BHT

(C)- Azodicarbonamide

(D)- Bleached Starch

119- Which one was established in 1963?

(A)- World Federation of Neurosurgical Societies

(B)- German Agency for Quality in Medicine

(C)- Doctors Reform Society of Australia

(D)- Indian Academy of Pediatrics

120- When red blood cells are destroyed earlier than normal it is ...

(A)- Empty Sella Syndrome

(B)- Hereditary Spherocytosis

(C)- Formaldeyde Poisoning

(D)- Oral-Facial-Digital Syndrome

(Chapter 8) Answers

106- B

107- C

108- C

109- B

110- A

111- D

112- B

113- B

114- D

115- C

116- B

117- B

118- A

119- D

120- B

(Chapter 9)

121- This is a fungal infection of the mouth.

(A)- Oral Thrush

(B)- Fox-Fordyce Disease

(C)- Homonymous Hemianopsia

(D)- Distal Humerus Fracture

122- Johnson & Johnson agreed to pay an $8.9 billion settlement over claims that its ___ based baby powder caused cancer.

(A)- Triclosan

(B)- Benzene

(C)- Talc

(D)- Parabeans

123- This is also called brittle bone disease.

(A)- Blue Diaper Syndrome

(B)- Malnutrition

(C)- Osteogensis Imperfecta

(D)- Acanthosis Nigricans

124- When tumors start in the womb related to pregnancy it is ...

(A)- Cerebrocostomandibular Syndrome

(B)- Parvovirus B19

(C)- Gestational Trophoblastic Disease

(D)- MELAS Syndrome

125- This was founded in 1989.

(A)- AIDS Research Alliance

(B)- Brain Injury Research Institute

(C)- Center for Global Infectious Disease Research

(D)- Pennington Biomedical Research Center

126- Which one is also known as metatarsophalangeal joint sprain?

(A)- Transverse Fracture

(B)- Otitis Media with Effusion

(C)- Turf Toe

(D)- Fungal Nail Infection

127- The median age at diagnosis is approximately 60 years old for this.

(A)- Sarcoidosis

(B)- Carbon Monoxide Poisoning

(C)- De Quervain's Tenosynovitis

(D)- Angioimmunoblastic T-Cell Lymphoma

128- This is a condition where a child is born with missing or underdeveloped chest muscles.

(A)- Triple-A Syndrome

(B)- Poland Syndrome

(C)- Northern Epilepsy Syndrome

(D)- Rh Deficiency Syndrome

129- Since 1954, this has been banned in the United States.

(A)- Bisphenol A

(B)- Coumarin

(C)- Perfluoralkyl Chemicals

(D)- Chromium-6

130- This is a disorder that is passed down through families. It causes bad cholesterol level to be very high.

(A)- Nontuberculous Mycobacterial Lung Disease

(B)- Familial Hypercholesterolemia

(C)- Tangier Disease

(D)- Pityriasis Rosea

131- This is a sensation of motion or spinning that is often described as dizziness.

(A)- Septic Emboli

(B)- Vertigo

(C)- Uncal Herniation

(D)- Asperger Syndrome

132- Patricia Resick is known for developing this.

(A)- Chemotherapy

(B)- Stem-cell Therapy

(C)- Electroconvulsive Therapy

(D)- Cognitive Processing Therapy

133- This is also known as Briquet's Syndrome.

(A)- Adjustment Disorder

(B)- Disruptive Mood Dysregulation Disorder

(C)- Somatization Disorder

(D)- Developmental Coordination Disorder

134- Which one is a disease that is associated with dysfunction of the proximal tubule of the kidney?

(A)- Howel-Evans Syndrome

(B)- Renal Fanconi Syndrome

(C)- Stockholm Syndrome

(D)- Cockayne Syndrome

135- Vitelliform macular dystrophy is known as ...

(A)- CNS Whipple Disease

(B)- Felty Syndrome

(C)- Goodpasture Syndrome

(D)- Best Disease

136- This disorder was originally described in 1981 by Cornelis Jakobs, Ph.D.

(A)- Heavy Metal Poisoning

(B)- Guanidinoacetate Methyltransferase Deficiency

(C)- Juberg-Marsidi Syndrome

(D)- Succinic Semialdehyde Dehydrogenase Deficiency

137- This is a rare congenital skeletal abnormality where a person has one shoulder blade that sits higher on the back than the other.

(A)- Limb Length Discrepancy

(B)- Sprengel's Deformity

(C)- Trismus Pseudocamptodactyly Syndrome

(D)- Osteochondritis Dissecans

138- This is an autoimmune condition that mostly affects males over 50.

(A)- Congenital Generalized Lipodystrophy

(B)- Ring Chromosome 18

(C)- VEXAS Syndrome

(D)- SYNGAP1-related Intellectual Disability

139- Which one is a neurological disorder in which a fluid-filled cyst (syrinx) forms within the spinal cord?

(A)- Syringomyelia

(B)- Ovotesticular Disorder of Sex Development

(C)- Medullary Sponge Kidney

(D)- Trichorhinophalangeal Syndrome Type II

140- This is caused by blood clots that completely or partially block blood flow from the liver.

(A)- Ciguatera Fish Poisoning

(B)- Budd Chiari Syndrome

(C)- Gestational Trophoblastic Disease

(D)- Holt Oram Syndrome

(Chapter 9) Answers

121- A

122- C

123- C

124- C

125- A

126- C

127- D

128- B

129- B

130- A

131- B

132- D

133- C

134- B

135- D

136- D

137- B

138- C

139- A

140- B

(Chapter 10)

141- Mucopolysaccharidosis type III is also known as ...

(A)- Underload Syndrome

(B)- Sanfilippo Syndrome

(C)- Insulin Resistance Syndrome

(D)- Reinstein-Taybi Syndrome

142- Since 1956, this has been permitted by the U.S. FDA.

(A)- Blue #1

(B)- Yellow 2G

(C)- FD&C Green 3

(D)- Citrus Red #2

143- Dyspepsia is also known as ...

(A)- Moyamoya Disease

(B)- Indigestion

(C)- Muscle Pain

(D)- Hypothermia

144- This was established on September 6, 2006.

(A)- National Center for Research Resources

(B)- Collaborative Study on the Genetics of Alcoholism

(C)- Ear Research Foundation

(D)- Janelia Research Campus

145- This most commonly affects the muscles that control the eyes and eyelids, facial expressions, chewing, swallowing, and speaking.

(A)- Myasthenia Gravis

(B)- Chronic Neutrophilic Leukemia

(C)- Sinonasal undifferentiated carcinoma

(D)- Longus Colli Muscle

146- Breathing smoke or coming into contact with contaminated soil exposes people to this and may cause cancer and may affect the eyes, kidneys, and liver.

(A)- Herbicide

(B)- Pesticide

(C)- Arsenic

(D)- Polycyclic Aromatic Hydrocarbons

147- This is a skin inflammation that is in part of the fatty layer of skin.

(A)- Condylomata Acuminata

(B)- Ribonucleic Acid

(C)- Acanthocheilonemiasis

(D)- Erythema Nodosum

148- Which one was founded in 1954?

(A)- American Society of Addiction Medicine

(B)- Royal College of Nursing

(C)- NPS MedicineWise

(D)- Hong Kong College of Physicians

149- This is an uncommon condition that affects the brain and nerves.

(A)- Marinesco-Sjögren Syndrome

(B)- Germinoma

(C)- Motor Neurone Disease

(D)- Adamantinoma

150- Which one is an inherited disease that affects a person's height, muscles, skeleton, genitals, and appearance of the face?

(A)- Richter's Transformation

(B)- Dehydroepiandrosterone

(C)- Aarskog Syndrome

(D)- Immunopathogenesis

151- This is a genetic disorder that causes people to have unusually long arms, legs, and fingers.

(A)- Marfan Syndrome

(B)- Juvenile Ossifying Fibroma

(C)- Von Hippel-Lindau Disease

(D)- Metastatic Carcinoma

152- When fluid fills a male's scrotum causing it to swell, it is ...

(A)- Undescended Testicles

(B)- Summer Penile Syndrome

(C)- Balanitis

(D)- Hydrocele

153- This is also known as tartrazine.

(A)- Caramel Coloring

(B)- Brown HT

(C)- Yellow #5

(D)- Yellow #6

154- Which one was established in 1994?

(A)- TAF Preventive Medicine Bulletin

(B)- Academic Emergency Medicine

(C)- European Journal of Cancer Prevention

(D)- Journal of Occupational and Environmental Medicine

155- This is a rare complication of pelvic inflammatory disease.

(A)- Vulvar Intraepithelial Neoplasia

(B)- Fitz-Hugh-Curtis Syndrome

(C)- Lymphogranuloma Venereum

(D)- Uterine Fibroids

(Chapter 10) Answers

141- B

142- D

143- B

144- D

145- A

146- D

147- D

148- A

149- C

150- C

151- A

152- D

153- C

154- B

155- B

(Chapter 11)

156- This is also called CN VIII.

(A)- Costocervical trunk

(B)- Vestibulocochlear nerve

(C)- Sphenomandibular ligament

(D)- Pterygopalatine ganglion

157- This is a mineral that occurs naturally in soil, water, and air that has been shown to prevent cavities and tooth decay.

(A)- Lead

(B)- Chlorine

(C)- Fluoride

(D)- Chloramine

158- This was first talked about in 1883.

(A)- Waldenström macroglobulinemia

(B)- Marcus Gunn Syndrome

(C)- Deafness-ichthyosis-keratitis Syndrome

(D)- River Blindness

159- Which one is also known as valley fever?

(A)- Proteinuria

(B)- Frostbite

(C)- Venous Thromboembolism

(D)- Coccidioidomycosis

160- This is a type of memory loss that occurs when you can't form new memories.

(A)- Branchiootorenal Spectrum Disorders

(B)- Exploding Head Syndrome

(C)- Anterograde Amnesia

(D)- Campomelic Syndrome

161- Chickenpox is associated with this.

(A)- Varicella

(B)- Mayer-Rokitansky-Küster-Hauser (MRKH) Syndrome

(C)- Uterine Atony

(D)- System Lupus Erythematosus

162- In 1991, Kimishige Ishizaka was appointed president and scientific director of ...

(A)- La Jolla Institute for Immunology

(B)- Miami Project to Cure Paralysis

(C)- National Wilms Tumor Study Group

(D)- Rush Alzheimer's Disease Center

163- This is a genetic condition that mainly affects the bones.

(A)- Camurati-Engelmann Disease

(B)- Thoracic Outlet Syndrome

(C)- Lipoma

(D)- Axenfeld-Rieger Syndrome

164- This is a type of arthritis that causes inflammation in the joints and ligaments of the spine.

(A)- Patellofemoral Pain Syndrome

(B)- Angioedema

(C)- Paraneoplastic Syndrome

(D)- Ankylosing Spondylitis

165- A chronic condition affecting the musculoskeletal system is ...

(A)- Intracranial Hematoma

(B)- Cerebral Small Vessel Disease

(C)- Encephalitis

(D)- Myofascial Pain Syndrome

166- From birth this causes many parts of the body to develop abnormally.

(A)- Lacunar Stroke

(B)- Noonan Syndrome

(C)- Deoxyhypusine Synthase Disorder

(D)- Primary Intestinal Lymphangiectasia

167- Which one is known as Black Urine Disease?

(A)- Vogt-Koyanagi-Harada Disease

(B)- Kernicterus

(C)- Hermansky-Pudlak Syndrome

(D)- Alkaptonuria

168- This is a rare disorder that mainly occurs in postmenopausal women.

(A)- Neurofibromatosis Type 1

(B)- Achard-Thiers Syndrome

(C)- Staphylococcus Aureus

(D)- Enterohemorrhagic E. coli

169- Which one is diagnosed in kids that become uncooperative and unusually angry?

(A)- Brief Psychotic Disorder

(B)- Oppositional Defiant Disorder

(C)- Capgras Delusion

(D)- Bilateral Vestibulopathy

170- This is a rare condition that usually starts with a tumor in your appendix.

(A)- Rhabdomyolysis

(B)- Ichthyosis Hystrix, Curth-Macklin Type

(C)- Pseudomyxoma Peritonei

(D)- Dent Disease

(Chapter 11) Answers

156- B

157- C

158- B

159- D

160- C

161- A

162- A

163- A

164- D

165- D

166- B

167- D

168- B

169- B

170- C

(Chapter 12)

171- This is a relatively common growth on the skin. It is a fast-growing, small-sized, benign skin tumor that originates in the hair follicles.

(A)- Keratoacanthoma

(B)- Intussusception

(C)- Xerostomia

(D)- Tularemia

172- This is a rare autosomal recessive genetic ciliary disorder characterized by situs inversus, chronic sinusitis, bronchiectasis, and infertility.

(A)- Iridocyclitis

(B)- Ehlers-Danlos Syndrome

(C)- Episcleritis

(D)- Kartagener Syndrome

173- Often caused by stones that block the tube leading from the gallbladder to the small intestine, is known as ...

(A)- Cytomegalovirus

(B)- Menorrhagia

(C)- Cholecystitis

(D)- Bradycardia

174- Which one is used to treat epilepsy?

(A)- Allopurinol

(B)- Gabapentin

(C)- Mounjaro

(D)- Revefenacin

175- Complete Blood Count (CBC) is also known as ...

(A)- Maximum Blood Count

(B)- Full Blood Count

(C)- Overall Blood Count

(D)- Final Blood Count

176- The medical term for itchy skin is ...

(A)- Seborrhea

(B)- Pruritus

(C)- Spondylosis

(D)- Pustules

177- Anogenital warts are also known as ...

(A)- Osteomyelitis

(B)- Laryngomalacia

(C)- UARS

(D)- Condyloma Acuminata

178- When your eyes gradually lose the ability to see things up close, it is ...

(A)- Post-concussion syndrome

(B)- Retronychia

(C)- Lichen planus

(D)- Presbyopia

179- This is considered a cure for ulcerative colitis.

(A)- Esophagectomy

(B)- Proctocolectomy

(C)- Diverticulum

(D)- Pericardum

180- Prolonged or repeated exposure of this causes kidney cancer.

(A)- Crystalline Silica

(B)- Ethylene Oxide

(C)- Trichloroethylene

(D)- Beryllium

181- It's estimated about 1 in every 25 boys are born with ...

(A)- Undescended Testicles

(B)- Childhood-Onset Fluency Disorder

(C)- Omphalocele

(D)- Congenital Limb Defect

182- This is a medicine that lowers cholesterol.

(A)- Ezetimibe

(B)- Simethicone

(C)- Naproxen

(D)- Ramdesivir

183- 38% of the population has this blood type, making it the most common.

(A)- A negative

(B)- B positive

(C)- AB negative

(D)- O positive

(184)- Allergy testing, and tuberculosis (TB) screening commonly have these injections.

(A)- Subcutaneous Injections

(B)- Intraosseous Injections

(C)- Intradermal Injections

(D)- Intramuscular Injections

(185)- Absence of the nipple and areola on a child's breast is ...

(A)- Microtia

(B)- Adolescence Syndrome

(C)- Congenital Athelia

(D)- Dilated Cardiomyopathy

(Chapter 12) Answers

171- A

172- D

173- C

174- B

175- B

176- B

177- D

178- D

179- B

180- C

181- A

182- A

183- D

184- C

185- C

(Chapter 13)

186- Which one doesn't have to do with the eye?

(A)- Morton neuroma

(B)- Paralytic strabismus

(C)- Bjerrum Scotoma

(D)- Schirmer's test

187- This is a rare condition of the nervous system that causes gradual damage to nerve cells in the brain.

(A)- Brain Stem Stroke

(B)- Frontotemporal dementia

(C)- HSV encephalitis

(D)- Multiple system atrophy

188- This is used alone or in combination with other medicines to treat brain tumors, Hodgkin's disease, and other kinds of cancer.

(A)- Mexiletine

(B)- Natalizumab

(C)- Infliximab

(D)- Lomustine

189- This is a condition in which urine flows backward from the bladder to one or both ureters and sometimes to the kidneys.

(A)- Hemiballismus

(B)- Vesicoureteral reflux

(C)- Tick paralysis

(D)- Inclusion Body Myositis

190- Which one causes people to express negative feelings and emotions subtly rather than directly?

(A)- Schizotypal Personality Disorder

(B)- Narcissistic Personality Disorder

(C)- Passive-Aggressive Personality Disorder

(D)- Avoidant Personality Disorder

191- Barium swallow is also called ...

(A)- Dialysis

(B)- Globulin Test

(C)- Esophagogram

(D)- Taste Bud

192- This is a condition in infants in which the bile ducts outside and inside the liver are scarred and blocked.

(A)- Biliary atresia

(B)- Transient Ischemic Attack

(C)- Bradykinesia

(D)- Myasthenia Gravis

193- What year did Dr. Jack Lapides at the University of Michigan, introduce the clean intermittent catheterization technique?

(A)- 1929

(B)- 1971

(C)- 1999

(D)- 2021

194- This is a rare but serious disease caused by a toxin (poison) that attacks the nervous system and causes paralysis in children and adults.

(A)- Botulism

(B)- Erosive gastritis

(C)- Juvenile Nasopharyngeal Angiofibroma

(D)- Phyllodes tumor

195- Age-related hearing loss is ...

(A)- Sturge-Weber Syndrome

(B)- Meningococcemia

(C)- Prader-Willi Syndrome

(D)- Presbycusis

196- Which one is a rare type of noncancerous (benign) brain tumor?

(A)- Analgesic Rebound Headache

(B)- Pseudotumor Cerebri

(C)- Brown-Sequard Syndrome

(D)- Craniopharyngiomas

197- This is a rare mood disorder. It causes emotional ups and downs, a milder form of bipolar disorder.

(A)- Alcoholic cerebellar degeneration

(B)- Corticobasal degeneration

(C)- Tardive Dyskinesia

(D)- Cyclothymia

198- This may be used to treat infections caused by susceptible bacteria, such as: Bone infections. Ear infections (e.g., otitis media) Skin infections.

(A)- Flurazepam

(B)- Cephalosporin

(C)- Dinoprostone

(D)- Echothiophate

199- A bacterial infection causing inflammation of the kidneys and is one of the most common diseases of the kidney is...

(A)- Necrosectomy

(B)- Fasciotomy

(C)- Acute Pyelonephritis

(D)- Acute coronary syndrome

200- This is also known as fainting.

(A)- Syncope

(B)- Meniere's Disease

(C)- Persistent Vegetative State

(D)- Parinaud Syndrome

(Chapter 13) Answers

186- A

187- D

188- D

189- B

190- C

191- C

192- A

193- B

194- A

195- D

196- D

197- D

198- B

199- C

200- A

(Final Thoughts)

I mentioned it in the beginning of the book about the importance of paying attention to the things we consume. I just wanted to share some things I try to pay attention to. Parents buy things for our sporting events. Beverages like Kool-Aid Jammers and Capri Sun Juice Pouches. With Kool-Aid Jammers, it has citric acid, high-fructose corn syrup, synthetic vitamins, artificial colors and flavors, and the list goes on. There was a recall on approximately 5,760 cases of Capri Sun, or a total of about 230,400 individual drink pouches, that were potentially contaminated with cleaning solution. So, there's that issue. But even without the contamination, the drinks are still unhealthy. It's high in sugar, has artificial sweeteners and flavors, doesn't have essential vitamins, and the list goes on. My kids have filtered water and make their own healthy smoothies and cold-pressed juice. We try to keep things as natural as possible.

After a tennis match, the coach wanted to take the kids to Dairy Queen for ice cream. You might be thinking, that seems harmless. Well, let's talk about that "ice cream." It's filled with additives and artificial flavor; the FDA considers Polysorbate 80 safe, but it can cause intestinal and digestive issues. Can alter the nutrient absorption of ionic minerals like potassium and calcium. Ice cream needs at least 10% milk fat. Carrageenan is used to help thicken the product and make up for the lack of milk and other natural things that keep ice cream pure. Carrageenan can lead to diabetes, heart diseases, digestive disorders, neurological disorders, and other chronic illnesses. So, things that may seem harmless, or every time you consider something a "cheat day" and let something slide just this one time, eventually it adds up. Trying your best to keep a healthy routine and not getting caught up in bad habits is your best bet.

I'm not against eating meat; I enjoy it! But the type of meat is important. Grass-fed, pasture-raised organic meat is ideal. Buying from companies that are certified or have a reputation for selling the right meat is what I encourage. Eating chicken, burgers, and pizza from most fast-food restaurants is usually a bad idea. I'm sure most people know it can be unhealthy, but I don't think most people realize how unhealthy it is or the actual things that are injected into the things on the menu. Just taking time to research and making a commitment to caring about what you eat, and drink is important. I know it can be expensive. I know it might not seem delicious. I know change can be hard. But making the necessary changes to your health can be better for you and the people you care about in the short and long term.

I also want to warn you about not just accepting what corporations slap on packaging. Just because something says it's healthy or they use the key buzz words doesn't mean it's true. It still takes awareness and research on your part to make sure it's true. It would be nice to go to the store and just grab something without having to worry about whether it's truly healthy or not. Unfortunately, in the United States, the FDA and others who are supposed to look out for the well-being of people rarely actually do it. They're willing to sell off their integrity to the highest bidder. I like that Europe takes health a lot more seriously and is willing to stand up to corporations when it comes to food and beverages. Look at the labels of products sold in the U.S. and those same products sold in Europe. You'll see that Europe won't allow many of the unhealthy things to be sold. In Europe and Latin America, some products have warning levels that let you know when something is deemed bad.

Maybe you'll think about some of the things I brought up if you're not already doing it. Hopefully, you also found this book helpful when learning new things about health. Sometimes the very complex trivia might not be as fun or interesting for some people.

(List of My Books)

10 Categories of Trivia

200 Mixed Trivia Questions

AWARDS AND HONORS TRIVIA

Black Trivia Book

Colleges and Universities Trivia

College Trivia Nights

Healthy Habits

Health and Medical Trivia

I'll Tell You Why I Do It

Let's Talk About Women's Basketball

Making Sacrifices

Men Are Victims Too

Men in Sports Trivia

Music Trivia Book

People in Films and Shows Trivia

Real-life Lessons

Reflecting on My Interactions with Strangers

Religion Trivia

Stories of Struggling Fathers, Broken Families, and a Broken System

My email: LanceCares@gmail.com